EMOTIONAL MASTERY
FOR ADULTS WITH
ASPERGERS

PRACTICAL TECHNIQUES TO WORK THROUGH

ANXIETY, ANGER AND DEPRESSION.

Mark Blakey and Leslie Burby

Copyright

© 2012 by Aspergers Test Site. All rights reserved. No part of this document may be reproduced or transmitted in any form or by any means, electronic, mechanical, photocopying, recording, or otherwise, without prior written permission of the Aspergers Test Site.

The authors of this book have written this as a guide of helpful suggestions. This book is not intended as a substitute for the medical advice of physicians. The reader should regularly consult a physician in matters relating to his/her health and particularly with respect to any symptoms that may require diagnosis or medical attention.

Thank you

Thank you for downloading our book. We hope that it gives you some valuable insights and tools that you can use in your life.

We would be really grateful if you could review the book on Amazon.com. We do appreciate you feedback and if you have suggestions about how this book could be improved please feel to drop us a line at info@AspergersTestSite.com

For more helpful information on Aspergers Syndrome you can subscribe to our newsletter at:
http://www.aspergerstestsite.com/aspergers-newsletter

Table of Contents

About the Authors

Mark G. Blakey

Mark Blakey is the founder of the Asperger's Test Site, which he set up following his own diagnosis with Asperger's. Moving away from a successful career in Information Technology, Mark had been inspired to change careers and work in the field of personal growth. Training extensively in Psychotherapy, he is now a member of the British Association of Counseling and Psychotherapy (BACP). Mark runs workshops to help groups of individuals work through emotional traumas and realize their potential as human beings.

Leslie A. Burby

Leslie Burby is the owner of <u>Tutoring and Learning Resources of CT</u>. She resides in CT with her husband and three kids. Her oldest daughter has Asperger's Syndrome. Before becoming a mother, Leslie tutored at private and public schools in addition to in-home tutoring. She attended Franklin Pierce College and Saint Joseph's University. Leslie spends most of her professional time writing about Asperger's Syndrome, education and topics revolving around the two. When she is not writing books or running her household, she enjoys reading, writing, baking, playing board games and going to the beach.

Preface

Following the creation of the Asperger's Test Site, we received a steady flow of questions from people seeking advice following their diagnosis. One of the things we noticed is that it is the emotional aspect of their lives' that they struggle with the most. Issues around anxiety, stress, anger and depression are quite common.

Most of the people asking questions are adults, who have suffered most of their life with an array of symptoms that they could not label, understand or work towards healing. It is only in the past 15 or 20 years that Asperger's Syndrome has come into public awareness. For the generation born before 1980, the condition was overlooked and those with Asperger's symptoms often encountered a struggle during their formative school years. They felt aware that something was different in the way they were relating, but were not sure exactly what these differences were.

Emotional awareness is not something that we are taught in school and it is rarely even understood by our parents. We live in a society where even those not in the Autistic Spectrum (Neuro-typical Individuals) suffer to some extent with emotional repression and its subsequent side effects. Is it then not surprising that most with Asperger's syndrome struggle to get the help, knowledge and understanding to live a healthy and happy life.

For this reason, we decided to write this book about emotional mastery. It is intended to give you a better understanding of the emotions that affect those living with Asperger's syndrome. In writing this book, we deemed first to identify what the problem areas are before looking for resolutions. While we could not cover every single emotion in this book, we have covered the ones that are most problematic. We hope you will gain a deeper insight by understanding the medical basis for your particular symptoms.

Along with each chapter we are going to suggest helpful techniques that you may find helpful in coming to terms with these conditions. Use them as a guide. We are all unique individuals and developing mastery in any area of our lives involves testing different techniques and determining what works best for us.

We hope this book will give you the tools and understanding you need to both master your emotions and master your life!

Chapter 1 Emotions

Our emotional system is a very fundamental part of our lives; however, this important aspect of our being is often overlooked. Tragically, emotional intelligence is not taught in school and frequently not by our parents or society. This leads to an inability to understand this driving force of our actions and behaviors.

Emotions trigger thoughts and physical responses in the body, both of which determine how we act.
Our long-term physical health is also affected by the emotions we experience on a regular basis. You may have noticed that you are most likely to get sick or suffer from physical ailments when you are stressed, anxious or unhappy.

What are emotions?

It is difficult to define the emotional system as one separate aspect of ourselves. It is a complex relationship, which occurs between our bodies and minds. Thoughts trigger emotions and emotions trigger thoughts. These in turn trigger our habitual patterns of reactions and behaviors.

We could write a long definition from the scientific community about the nature of emotions but in essence, emotions are what make us human. They define our subjective conscious experience of life.

Here is a brief overview of emotions, if you would like a detailed explanation of the emotional system, we recommend you read Candace Pert's book entitled "Molecules of Emotion."

The body mind recognizes specific physical and emotional states through the stimulation of receptors, which are attached to cells in the body. Receptors are sensing mechanisms, which await the insertion of a chemical key. These chemical keys are called ligands. Receptors ignore all but a ligand made to fit. Hence, the response of a cell is different depending on which ligand is binding. Every cell in the body contains hundreds of thousands of receptors.

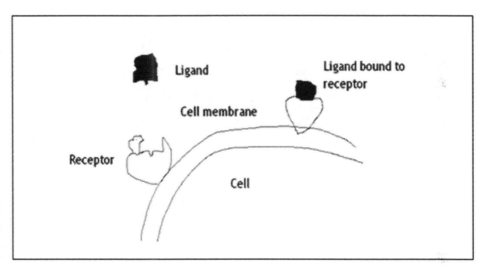

Figure 1: Diagram showing how ligands connect with receptors located on the edge of the cell membrane

Once the ligand binds to the receptor it triggers a chain reaction of biochemical events such as: blood flow, heart rate, steroid production and cell division.

There are several types of ligands:

- o Steroids
- o Neurotransmitters

o   Peptides

Peptides or neuropeptides (peptides associated with brain activity) are related to the various emotional states. These include anger, fear, disgust, sadness, anticipation, joy, acceptance and surprise. The manifestations of these emotions become apparent in bodily and facial expressions that are independent of social conditioning. It has been proven, for example, that the facial expression for anger is the same between an Italian and an Eskimo.

Identifying emotions

One of the first steps to attaining emotional mastery is to begin to understand the emotions that are present within us in each moment. So many of us are unaware of what we are feeling, causing us to act unconsciously in reaction to the physical sensations that occur in the body when emotions are experienced.

When we understand that we are feeling a certain emotion, we begin to choose to act in a different way. A way that leads us towards fulfillment rather than the downward spiral of negative emotions that can occur when we don't know any other way of dealing with situations.

One of the main ways that you can identify the feelings that exist within you, is through your body. All emotions have a physical effect in the body and this is true of positive emotions like joy and love as well as what we deem negative emotions, like anger or anxiety. When we feel elated with joy, our body feels loose and light and we cannot help but smile. If we feel angry our body becomes tense, we often frown or clench our jaws and teeth.

While we can experience a full spectrum of emotions, you will experience some on a more regular basis. See which emotions you identify with the most from the list below. You may find it useful to write down the physical sensations that you experience when you feel that particular emotion. Then the next time you experience that physical sensation it will help you to recognize the emotion.

- Fear
- Anger
- Sadness
- Joy
- Disgust
- Trust
- Anticipation
- Surprise

As well as the primary emotions listed above, there are a whole range of other feelings that are included within the human conscious.

- Absorbed
- Accepting
- Accommodating
- Accomplished
- Adaptable
- Adversarial
- Aggressive
- Agreeable
- Alert
- Altruistic
- Analytical
- Annoyed
- Antagonistic

- Anxious
- Approved of
- Arrogant
- Ashamed
- Authentic
- Balanced
- Beautiful
- Belligerent
- Bereft
- Bitter
- Bored
- Brave
- Broken down
- Bullied
- Calm
- Chaotic
- Cheerful
- Cold
- Compassionate
- Competitive
- Conceited
- Condemned
- Confident
- Conflicted
- Confused
- Conservative
- Content
- Controlled
- Controlling
- Cooperative
- Courageous
- Cowardly

- Creative
- Critical
- Cruel
- Curious
- Defeated
- Deluded
- Demanding
- Dependent
- Depressed
- Desperate
- Destitute
- Destructive
- Detached
- Dignified
- Disconnected
- Discouraged
- Disgusted
- Dominated
- Dominating
- Eccentric
- Ecstatic
- Egocentric
- Egotistical
- Empathic
- Empowered
- Envious
- Erratic
- Excited
- Expressive
- Extroverted
- Fair
- Faithful

- Fearful
- Frightened
- Frustrated
- Glad
- Good
- Grateful
- Greedy
- Grieving
- Guilty
- Happy
- Harmonizing
- Hatred
- Helpful
- Helpless
- Hesitant
- Hopeless
- Idealistic
- Ignorant
- Impatient
- Important
- Impoverished
- Impulsive
- Indifferent
- Individualistic
- Inert
- Insecure
- Insensitive
- Inspired
- Interested
- Intolerant
- Introspective
- Invulnerable

- Irresponsible
- Irritated
- Isolated
- Jealous
- Joyful
- Judged
- Judgmental
- Lazy
- Likable
- Lively
- Lonely
- Lost
- Loved
- Loving
- Mad
- Manipulated
- Manipulative
- Mediating
- Miserable
- Mistrusting
- Moody
- Moral
- Negative
- Noble
- Obsessed
- Open
- Panicked
- Paranoid
- Passionate
- Passive
- Peaceful
- Pleased

- Poor
- Possessive
- Powerful
- Practical
- Preoccupied
- Proud
- Punished
- Punishing
- Purposeful
- Rage
- Reactionary
- Reclusive
- Rejected
- Repressed
- Resentful
- Resigned
- Resistant
- Responsible
- Ridiculous
- Righteous
- Ruthless
- Sad
- Sadistic
- Secretive
- Selfish
- Self-accepting
- Self-condemning
- Self-defeating
- Self-destructive
- Self-hatred
- Self-obsessed
- Self-pity

- Self-sabotaging
- Sensitive
- Serene
- Shamed
- Shut-down
- Shy
- Sorry
- Stable
- Stimulated
- Stubborn
- Superiority
- Timid
- Tolerant
- Unconcerned
- Understanding
- Unforgiving
- Unhappy
- Unresponsive
- Untrusting
- Vain
- Vengeance
- Vicious
- Victimized
- Violent
- Visionary
- Well-meaning
- Wise
- Withdrawn
- Worthy

Chapter 2 Anxiety and Stress

Anxiety and stress appear to be the emotions that most adults with Asperger's suffer from the most.

The words anxiety and stress are often used together or interchangeably, so we will clarify the meaning of each word. Although both feelings are caused by the fight-or-flight response, (a reaction of the sympathetic nervous system that increases the body's adrenaline and cortisol), they contain many differences. Stress comes from something, usually an event or person, which causes you to feel frustrated. Whereas anxiety invokes feelings of fear and does not necessarily, need a stressor.

While stress is not considered a mental illness, anxiety that lasts six months or more is deemed a mental disorder. Of course, a prolonged amount of stress can lead to an anxiety disorder. The anxiety disorders that mainly effect adults with Asperger's are: panic disorder, obsessive-compulsive disorder (OCD), social phobia (or social anxiety disorder) and generalized anxiety disorder (GAD).

According to National Institute of Mental Health (NIMH), the following anxiety disorders exist within adults with Asperger's:

1. Panic Disorder
2. Obsessive Compulsive Disorder (OCD)
3. Social Anxiety Disorder / Social Phobia
4. Generalized Anxiety Disorder (GAD)

Panic Disorder:

Those who suffer with panic disorder have sudden and repeated attacks of fear that can last for several minutes, although sometimes symptoms may last longer. These incidents of extended fear are called panic attacks. Panic attacks are characterized by a fear of impending disaster or of losing control, even when there is no actual danger. A person may also have a strong physical reaction to external circumstances, experiencing symptoms, which may feel like a heart attack. Panic attacks can occur at any time; many people with panic disorder worry about and dread the possibility of having another attack.

A person with panic disorder may become discouraged and feel ashamed because he or she cannot carry out normal routines like going to the grocery store or driving. Having panic disorder can also interfere with one's school or work. Panic disorder often begins in the late teens or early adulthood. More women than men have panic disorder; although not everyone who experiences panic attacks will go on to develop panic disorder.

Many people can experience a panic attack without further episodes or complications. There is little reason to worry if you have had just one or two attacks. However, some people who have experienced panic attacks can go on to develop panic disorder. Panic disorder is characterized by repeated panic attacks combined with major changes in behavior or persistent anxiety over having further attacks.

Panic Disorder Symptoms

You may be suffering from panic disorder if you:

- Experience frequent, unexpected panic attacks that are not related to a specific situation.

- Worry excessively about having another panic attack.
- Are behaving differently because of the panic attacks such as avoiding places where you have previously experienced an attack.

While a single panic attack may only last a few minutes, the effects of the experience can leave a lasting imprint. If you have panic disorder, the recurrent panic attacks take an emotional toll. The memory of the intense fear and terror that you felt during the attacks can negatively affect your self-confidence and cause serious disruption to your everyday life. Eventually, this leads to the following panic disorder symptoms:

- **Anticipatory anxiety** – Instead of feeling relaxed and your usual self in between panic attacks, you feel anxious and tense. This anxiety stems from a fear of having future panic attacks. This "fear of fear" is present most of the time, and can be extremely disabling.
- **Phobic avoidance** – You begin to avoid certain situations or environments. This avoidance may be based on the belief that the situation you are avoiding caused a previous panic attack. You may avoid places where escape would be difficult or help would be unavailable if you had a panic attack. Taken to its extreme, phobic avoidance becomes *agoraphobia*.

Obsessive Compulsive Disorder (OCD)

Almost everyone double checks things in certain situations. For example, you might double check to make sure the stove or iron has been switched off before leaving the house. People with OCD feel the need to unnecessarily check things or perform routines and rituals repeatedly. They also think certain thought patterns continuously.

The thoughts and rituals associated with OCD cause distress and get in the way of daily life. These frequent upsetting thoughts are called obsessions. In an attempt to control these repetitive thoughts, a person will feel an overwhelming urge to repeat certain rituals or behaviors called compulsions. People with OCD are unable to control these obsessions and compulsions.

OCD Symptoms

For many people, OCD starts during childhood or the teenage years. Most people are diagnosed at around 19 years old. Symptoms of OCD may come and go and become better or worse at different times. The majority of people with obsessive-compulsive disorder (OCD) have both obsessions and compulsions, but some people experience just one or the other.

There are a number of thought patterns common to OCD, including:

- Fear of becoming contaminated by germs and dirt or contaminating others
- Fear of causing harm to yourself or others
- Intrusive sexually explicit or violent thoughts and images
- Excessive focus on religious or moral ideas
- Fear of losing or not having at hand things you might need
- Order and symmetry: the idea that everything must line up "just right"
- Superstitions: excessive attention to something considered lucky or unlucky

For a person with OCD, these thoughts can often lead to certain compulsive behaviors, which may include.

- Excessive double-checking of things, such as locks, appliances, and switches

- Repeatedly checking in on loved ones to make sure they are safe
- Counting, tapping, repeating certain words or doing other senseless things to reduce anxiety
- Spending a lot of time washing or cleaning
- Ordering or arranging things "just so"
- Praying excessively or engaging in rituals triggered by religious fear
- Accumulating junk such as old newspapers or empty food containers

Social Phobia/Social Anxiety Disorder:

Social phobia is a strong fear of being judged by others and experiencing feelings of embarrassment. This fear can be so strong that it gets in the way of attending work or school and doing other everyday things. Everyone has felt anxious or embarrassed at one time or another. For example, meeting new people or giving a public speech can make many people nervous, but those with social phobia worry excessively about these events and other situations for weeks before they happen.

People with social phobia are afraid of performing simple tasks in front of other people. For example, they might be afraid to eat or drink in front of other people or use a public restroom. Most people who have social phobia know that they do not need be as afraid as they are, but they are unable to control their fear. Sometimes, they end up avoiding places or events where they think they might have to do something that will embarrass them. For some people, social phobia is a problem only in certain situations, while others have symptoms in almost any social situation.

Social phobia usually starts during one's youth. A doctor can diagnose social phobia if the person has had symptoms for at least six months. Without treatment, social phobia can last for many years, even a lifetime.

Social Phobia symptoms

The symptoms of Social Phobia can be divided into emotional, physical and behavioral aspects.

Emotional symptoms:

- Excessive self-consciousness and anxiety in everyday social situations
- Intense worry for days, weeks or even months before an upcoming social situation
- Extreme fear of being watched or judged by others, especially people you do not know
- Fear that you will act in ways that that will embarrass or humiliate yourself
- Fear that others will notice that you are nervous

Physical symptoms:

- Red face or blushing
- Shortness of breath
- Upset stomach, nausea (i.e. butterflies)
- Trembling or shaking (including shaky voice)
- Racing heart or tightness in chest
- Sweating or hot flashes
- Feeling dizzy or faint

Behavioral symptoms:

- Avoiding social situations to a degree that limits your activities or disrupts your life
- Staying quiet or hiding in the background in order to escape notice and embarrassment
- A need to always bring a friend along with you wherever you go
- Drinking before social situations in order to soothe your nerves

Generalized Anxiety Disorder (GAD):

Most of us worry about things like health, money or family problems, but people with GAD are extremely worried about these and many other issues, even when there is little or no reason to worry. They can feel very anxious about just getting through the day. They fear things will always go badly. At times, this excessive worrying prevents people with GAD from carrying out everyday tasks.

GAD develops slowly. It often starts during the teen years or young adulthood. Symptoms may get better or worse at different times, and often become worse during times of stress.

People with GAD may visit a doctor many times before they find out they have this disorder. They attend their doctors for treatment for headaches or trouble falling asleep, which can be symptoms of GAD but they do not always get the help they need right away. It may take the doctor some time to correctly diagnose GAD, as the symptoms can point to various ailments.

Symptoms of generalized anxiety disorder (GAD)

The symptoms of generalized anxiety disorder (GAD) fluctuate. You may notice that they become worse at different times of the day, or that you experience good or bad days in general. While stress does not cause generalized anxiety disorder, it can make the symptoms worse. Not everyone with generalized anxiety disorder have the same symptoms, although most people with GAD experience a combination of a number of the following emotional, behavioral and physical symptoms.

Emotional

- Constant worries running through your head
- Feeling like your anxiety is uncontrollable; there is nothing you can do to stop the worrying
- Intrusive thoughts about things that make you anxious; you try to avoid thinking about them, but you cannot
- An inability to tolerate uncertainty; you need to know what is going to happen in the future
- A pervasive feeling of apprehension or dread

Behavioral

- Inability to relax, enjoy quiet time, or time alone
- Difficulty concentrating or focusing on things
- Putting things off because you feel overwhelmed
- Avoiding situations that make you anxious

Physical

- Feeling tense; having muscle tightness or body aches
- Having trouble falling asleep or staying asleep because your mind will not be quieted
- Feeling edgy, restless or jumpy
- Stomach problems, nausea, diarrhea

Causes of Anxiety

The majority of adults with Asperger's suffer with anxiety. Ryan Rivera of www.calmclinic.com, an expert on Asperger's Syndrome and anxiety estimates a 70% anxiety rate in people with Asperger's in comparison to 18% of individuals not on the Autism Spectrum.

There are many speculations as to why people with Asperger's have an increased risk of developing an anxiety disorder. It is usually a variety of contributing factors. Some people believe anxiety disorders are genetic in certain cases; in others' the disorder is thought to be a direct result of their upbringing and life circumstances. In addition, the lack of awareness regarding Asperger's before 1944 did not help the added feeling of anxiety that sufferers endured not understanding why they felt different.

Since people with Asperger's are blessed, or some might see it as cursed, with an amazing memory, it is common to vividly remember painful past experiences; this can often lead to the development of a social phobia, or in rare cases, PTSD −post traumatic stress disorder. PTSD occurs when a person suffers a severe traumatic event, which is emotionally scarring, leaving the person with flashbacks, frightening thoughts and nightmares. Please note that PTSD is not the result of Asperger's, it is the result of a terrifying and traumatic event.

Triggers are environmental factors that cause the body's adrenaline levels to increase, creating anxiety. Many Aspergian triggers are sensory related however; a panic attack can be triggered by various circumstances and occurrences. Everyone has different sensitivities, so it is important to pay attention to what affects you specifically; become aware of the situations and circumstances that trigger your panic attacks. Some people find it helpful to record a log of what was happening before, at the beginning, and during the anxiety attack to pinpoint triggers.

- Do loud sounds affect you?
- Does fluorescent lighting affect you?
- Do smells like scented candles or extremely fragrant perfume affect you?
- Does touch, soft or firm, affect you?

For others, triggers are not sensory related but a result of being uncertain. There is a great comfort for people with Asperger's in knowing what will come next; routines are often extremely important in providing a sense of security. Unfortunately, not everything always goes as planned. You can get a flat tire, the weather can change or people get sick, all which can lead to cancellations and adjustments in scheduling. Learning how to adjust and cope with adaptations can be extremely helpful and useful.

Chapter 3 Dealing with Anxiety

There are various ways to try to deal with anxiety. In this chapter, we will discuss different techniques in anxiety management. The techniques have been broken down into sections to help you find and navigate the strategies that are best suited to you. The type of anxiety disorder you have, will greatly determine which kind of technique will be the most beneficial.

Recognizing Triggers

One of the primary techniques for dealing with anxiety and panic attacks is recognizing your triggers. Triggers are any kind of stimuli that lead to a bout of anxiety. By understanding and recognizing the triggers, one can begin to avoid the onset of anxiety by avoiding or behaving differently around certain events.

By understanding and recognizing your triggers, you can develop strategies to avoid the onset of anxiety; this can be achieved by instigating changes in behavior and thought patterns around certain events. Once you recognize a trigger, you can move away from a situation until you feel calm and in control again, before a full-blown panic attack occurs.

There are two types of stimuli: external and internal.

External stimuli include anything that your senses can perceive in your external environment. Examples may include:

- Social gatherings

- Public transport
- Workplace
- Dating
- Types of events
- Certain smells
- Changes in temperature in the room
- Changes in lighting
- Noises or a change in the way things sound
- Strange tastes

Internal stimuli include events that happen inside one's self. Sometimes, these stimuli are not easy to detect. These may include:

- Thoughts
- Memories
- Emotions
- Dehydration
- Consumption of caffeine
- Skipping meals
- Bodily sensations such as a skipped heartbeat or stomach ache

Caffeine, in particular, is a common trigger for the onset of anxiety. It is worth correlating the times you experience anxiety to your daily caffeine intake. While coffee is a common factor, we are all unique and though the list may give you some insight, it is important to develop your own personal list of triggers, through personal observation. It is often helpful to keep a journal. Every time you realize you are encountering anxiety, make a note of what you had been thinking, doing and feeling when the onset of the anxiety began.

Many experts suggest writing down what affects you emotionally; charting your triggers is a great place to start. If you pinpoint that your triggers are mostly thought related, then it will help to write down your thoughts. Keep a small notepad with you and jot down what you were thinking prior to feeling anxious. This can show you a pattern of thinking that triggers your panic attacks, giving you a starting point for positive change. Some people find that writing down their thoughts onto paper are enough to expel them from their mind and prevent the attack.

After your panic attack, think back and try to remember all the details. You can create your own chart or make copies of the one provided in this book. Store your charts so that you have a detailed history of your panic attacks allowing you to create a strategic plan of action to combat further attacks. Date each document and record the location where the panic attack happened. This way you can observe if certain places like the grocery store or certain times of day are triggers for you.

Trigger Chart

Date: _____ Time: _____

Location: _____

Question	Answer
What was I thinking? Were you feeling stressed about bills, worried about something in particular or angry with someone?	
Was I thinking of the past? Was there a certain memory that you were thinking of?	

What emotions was I feeling? Stress, Worry, Fear, Doubt, etc.	
Did I have a "bodily sensation?" Did your heart skip? Did you have a headache or a stomachache?	
What did it smell like? Did I get a whiff of a strong odor? Was someone wearing a potent perfume? Was someone smoking near you?	
Was there a change in temperature? Was I too hot or too cold?	
How was the lighting? Was it too bright? Was it too dark? Were there florescent light bulbs?	
What did I hear? Were there many sounds all at once? Was there a sudden sound?	
Did you have a "funny taste in your mouth?"	

Did something visually affect you? Did a color or image that triggered a memory?	

Addressing Triggers

Once you figure out what your triggers are you can start to address them. Look for alternatives for your triggers, for example, in the movie, "My name is Khan" the main character's trigger was the color yellow. In the beginning of the movie, he has a panic attack whenever he sees the color yellow; however, later in the movie, he is able to turn away from the person wearing the color, allowing the feelings to subside. Equally, if you have a sensitivity to light, such as the florescent lighting in supermarkets, try wearing sunglasses inside or try to avoid that particular store altogether. Get creative in your approach to deviating from your triggers before an attack occurs.

If you cannot go to the grocery store, try using an online service like Peapod for grocery deliveries in the States. You can use Tesco or Waitrose if you live in the U.K.

Another alternative is to ask a family member or neighbor to do your shopping for you. Perhaps you can offer to tend to one of their chores in exchange. Another possibility is the option to hire an errand runner. There are many online services to choose from. You can check availability of an errand runner to carry out tasks such as grocery shopping, pharmacy runs, gift shopping, drop-off and pick-up dry cleaning, post office and banking. If you feel you have tried all other possibilities to prevent your attacks to no avail, it may be worth considering these options.

Some great sites in the U.S. are Errand Runner USA and Best Friend Errand, with prices averaging between $25-$30 dollars an hour or per errand (please check sites for specific rates).

Some great errand sites in the U.K. are My Errand Runner and Errands Plus with prices averaging from €9 to €20 depending on the service (please view sites for specific rates).

Give whoever is doing your shopping a specific list of items you require, give alternative options if the item is not available. Be specific about brand and item size, e.g. 40 oz. of the cheapest peanut butter available or 40 oz. of Jiffy's Smooth Peanut Butter and instructions if Jiffy is not in stock. Provide coupons if you use them. It may seem tedious at first, but if you use the same person to regularly shop for you, they will quickly learn your likes, dislikes and approved alternative items.

Whatever your triggers are, become creative and find alternatives to make your everyday life less stressful.

Affirmations

Another suggestion is to turn your worries into affirmations. Firstly, write down your worries, from these negative statements, create affirming statements, which are the direct opposite of the worry.

Worry: I worry about getting a panic attack on the bus

Affirmation: I am calm and safe and enjoy using the bus.

Negative self-scripts are beliefs, statements and self-images that you believe to be true about yourself, which affect your everyday actions and thoughts. Everyone has his or her own negative self-scripts. For adults with Asperger's the negative self-scripts usually originate from growing up in a society that was oblivious to the term "Asperger's Syndrome." Since diagnosis of Asperger's was not possible until 1994, many people encountered misdiagnosis and were subsequently mistreated.

Many people with Asperger's are familiar with being bullied and judged by Neuro-typicals. For instance, it is the norm for people with Asperger's to be clumsy due to a dysfunctional vestibular and proprioceptive system, which makes it difficult to regulate body movement and know where your body is in space. However, proprioception is still not common knowledge today, resulting in people without autism awareness to be judgmental of this invisible disability. Negative language has a tendency to linger in the mind and leave us with negative views of ourselves.

In order to rid yourself of negative self-scripts, you must first narrow down which ones you possess and replace them with positive self-scripts by creating affirmations.

"I am" -a statement of who you are.

This is a positive affirmation of a real state of being that exists in you. You can achieve a full list of "I am" statements by taking a personal positive inventory of your attributes, strengths, talents and competencies. 'I am' is one of the most powerful statements you can say; this is what determines your current realities. Notice if this is true in your life. What do you most often say to yourself or others? This becomes true for you.

Notice what happens when you drop those statements and replace them with positive 'I am' statements. Your emotions change when you change the way you express yourself.

Examples include:

- I am competent--I am energetic
- I am strong--I am enthusiastic

- I am intelligent--I am relaxed
- I am beautiful--I am joyful
- I am a good person--I am trusting
- I am caring--I am generous
- I am loving--I am courageous
- I am smart--I am forgiving
- I am creative--I am open
- I am talented--I am sharing

"I can"--a statement of your potential.

This is a positive affirmation of your ability to accomplish goals. It is a statement of your belief in your power to grow, to change and to help yourself. "I can" statements are created after you develop a set of short-term (3 to 6 months) goals. These short-term goals can be steps leading to larger goals. Examples include:

- I can lose weight--I can grow
- I can stop smoking--I can heal
- I can handle my children--I can let go of guilt
- I can gain self-confidence--I can let go of fear
- I can take risks--I can change
- I can be a winner--I can be positive
- I can be strong--I can be a problem solver
- I can pass calculus--I can handle my own problems
- I can laugh and have fun--I can be honest with my feelings
- I can be assertive--I can let go of being compulsive
- I can control my temper--I can succeed

Create positive affirmations of the areas you would like to change, based on the original list of worries that you experience. It must be a positive statement in the present tense, involving an emotion. Affirmations work because your sub conscious believes what you tell it and proceeds to attract experiences and feelings that match your request. Like attracts like. If you are constantly telling yourself, I am afraid of social events', I do not like parties, 'I hate travelling on the bus', I feel angry/sad/stressed etc., then that is what you will experience.

Choose one dilapidating worry that you have, work avidly on switching your belief by noticing when you are expressing this pattern and switching it immediately to your new positive affirmation. – I am in control of my emotions. I enjoy attending some parties. I allow my emotions to subside and feel good again.

It is when you dedicate to this new pattern of thinking that you will reap the rewards and know the value of positive affirmations. It is important to note that if you only use the affirmations for a few minutes a day and then resort back to your negative beliefs, you will be giving back the power to those beliefs and continue to create the feelings of fear, anxiety and stress that they are currently creating.

Dedication is required if change is to take place, affirmations need to replace your old thought patterns. If you say the affirmations with pure faith that they are true, with joy and gratitude in your heart, you will succeed.

- I like myself better each day.
- I gain emotional strength each day.
- I lose weight each day. – I enjoying taking good care of my body
- I feel great smoking less each day.
- I give others responsibility for their lives today.
- I take pride in being responsible for my feelings and behaviors.
- I grow emotionally stronger each day.
- I enjoy smiling at my customers and spreading some joy.
- I am confident about offering my comments in class.

- I praise my children today.
- I feel good things about me today.
- I sleep easily tonight.
- I release emotions that no longer serve me.
- I face my fears courageously today.
- I take on only what I can handle today.
- I take care of me today.
- I challenge myself to change today.
- I manage my time better today.
- I handle my finances wisely today.
- I take a risk to grow today.

The daily use of these "I" statements is another form of self-affirmation designed to counter negative self-concept. It can result in a positive attitude; optimism and can motivate you toward emotional growth and progress.

Post your positive affirmations in visible places such as on your bathroom mirror, car dashboard, desk and refrigerator so you are reminded constantly of your new way of being and instilling a new positive emotional state. Write them in your diary, use as screen savers on your computer. Chant them in your mind as you drive or walk to work; say them out loud as you shower or other times when alone. This also prevents the worrisome thoughts from entering your head. Whenever you are facing a situation that usually causes you concern, begin an inner dialogue of positive affirmations instead of negative self-talk. In time, this will become your new belief and subsequent pattern of behavior.

Do not dwell on the past – List the future

It is imperative that you do not dwell on past events or circumstances, instead envision your future as you would like it to be. Do not let fear or past bad experiences stop you from living your life to the fullest. If you fear failure because you were ridiculed the last time you did not achieve success, try to see this past situation as a lesson now learned and acknowledge that the past does not determine the future.

If you fear failure due to being ridiculed in the past (when you did not achieve the success you expected), learn from that situation. Is there any such thing as failure? Could 'failure' be a sign that you need to change course, to look at the situation from a different angle or go in an entirely new direction? Create a plan of action when you want to undertake a new challenge. Foresee the possible obstacles and be prepared for the probability that obstacles may occur: develop a plan B, should these obstacles present themselves. Being prepared for challenging obstacles will help alleviate the stress and anxiety that accompanies these events. Knowing in advance that things can deviate from the plan is a good belief system to develop, to assist you in dealing with the inevitability of the change. Create an affirmation such as, "I easily and effortlessly adjust my direction when circumstances change."

I try to remind myself of Thomas Edison, one of my favorite inventors. Thomas Edison did not succeed in his first ten thousand attempts at inventing the light bulb, but when asked why he continued after his many failed attempts he replied, "I have not failed. I have just found 10,000 ways that will not work." So if something does not go as planned, find the lesson in every mistake and view it as moving one step closer to success.

It can be helpful to write down the goals that you would like to achieve and then take steps towards achieving those goals. If you set goals that are too high and then do not achieve them or become overwhelmed, it can bring on anxiety. However if we know what we want to achieve, we can create mini-goals towards that major desire. Setting small intermediate goals enables us to feel a sense of accomplishment when we achieve something that is attainable.

Some examples of this include:

Final Goal	Intermediate Attainable Goal
Becoming Vice President of the company	Getting promoted (each promotion can be one step towards VP)
Being independently wealthy	Take a step to be more financially responsible i.e. saving 10% of income, reducing the amount spent on magazines etc.
Be empathetic	Learn about empathy and some strategies and implement one at a time
Get married	Go on a date and work towards getting to know another person

Allow yourself time to make personal improvements. Being independently wealthy would be great; however, this goal must be broken down into smaller steps. You can set a goal to save or invest money each week. If you can manage to save a certain amount regularly each week, then you can increase the amount you save in the following weeks. Eventually you can look into investment options, which could then lead to eventual wealth.

Herbs

For many, natural herbs have provided a successful, natural way to ease anxiety. Some can be mildly sedative, so please read all instructions carefully. Herbs come in various forms, as herbal teas, pills, or powder form if you have sensitivity to the taste.

- **Passionflower**. Passionflower has been used for hundreds of years as a natural anxiety reliever and for insomnia. In 2001, a study showed that it was as effective as a popular anti-anxiety medication.

- **Valerian root**. Used for centuries as both a sleeping aid and as an aid for anxiety, many people rely on valerian root for relief.

- **Chamomile**. A popular tea, drinking chamomile will help reduce anxiety.

- **Kava Kava**. This plant from the South Pacific is frequently used to treat anxiety. However, those with liver problems should avoid using this herb.

- **St. John's Wort**. Used for centuries, this herb helps combat anxiety and depression, as well as relieving muscle aches and reducing inflammation.

- **Verbena**. Also known as wild hyssop or vervain, this herb is often used to help those suffering from anxiety and depression.

- **Skullcap**. Help your nervous tension subside by trying skullcap as a tea or in one of its many other forms.

- **Cowslip** ((Primula officinalis), is one of the most widely used medicinal herbs with beneficial effects over the human body. For anxiety, it is best in the form of tea.

- **Lemon balm**. Lemon balm helps reduce anxiety, especially when used with other calming herbs such as chamomile.

- **Hops**. Used to help cure anxiety and restlessness, hops are generally combined with passionflower, chamomile, or valerian root.

Cognitive Behavioral Therapy

Many psychologists highly recommend cognitive behavioral therapy, CBT, for adults with Asperger's Syndrome. Always check the practitioner's credentials and qualifications before embarking on a course of therapy, choosing a licensed and experienced professional. It is advisable to find a therapist that is knowledgeable about adults with Asperger's. Cognitive Behavioral Therapy, by a licensed and experienced psychologist, is highly recommended for all anxiety disorders.

There are different types of Cognitive Behavioral Therapy. Exposure Therapy, also known as systematic desensitization, is a type of Cognitive Behavioral Therapy that helps people face their fears by **slowly** desensitizing them from the fear.

There is CBT Group therapy that is helpful for conquering social fears and can help adults with Asperger's learn forms of nonverbal communication such as how to make eye contact. Another CBT approach is "thought-stopping," which helps people with OCD to be aware of when they are obsessing, so they can stop the obsessive thought pattern by doing an action such as yelling out, "STOP!", or using an alternative, quieter method of distraction such as snapping a rubber band on their wrist.

Four Steps for Conquering Symptoms of Obsessive-Compulsive Disorder (OCD)

Psychiatrist Jeffrey Schwartz, author of *Brain Lock: Free Yourself from Obsessive-Compulsive Behavior*, offers the following four steps for dealing with OCD:

RELABEL – Recognize that the intrusive obsessive thoughts and urges are the result of OCD. For example, train yourself to say:

- "I am completely aware that my hands are clean. I am just having an obsession that my hands are dirty."
- "I am completely aware that my hands are clean. I am having a compulsive urge to wash my hands"
- "My hands are clean. I am allowing this OCD compulsive thought to pass. I am in control of my thoughts and behavior. I enjoy recognizing the signs and changing direction"

REATTRIBUTE – Realize that the intensity and intrusiveness of the thought or urge that is caused by OCD; it is probably related to a biochemical imbalance in the brain. Tell yourself: "It is not my true belief—it is my OCD,"

Use these to remind you that OCD thoughts and urges are not meaningful, but are false messages from the brain and not reflective of what you truly believe to be true.

REFOCUS – Work around the OCD thoughts by focusing your attention on something else, at least for a few minutes. Do something completely different. Say to yourself, "I am experiencing a symptom of OCD. I am changing to a positive behavior."

REVALUE – Do not take the OCD thought at face value. It is not significant in itself. Tell yourself, "That's just my OCD obsession. It has no meaning. That is just my brain.

Other strategies

In the chapter, "Emotional Mastery", you will find an array of positive strategies and techniques relevant to all aspects of emotional health, which will assist you to positive change.

Chapter 4 - Anger Management

One of the most difficult issues for people with Asperger's is recognizing one's feelings, which is why most, if not all, struggle with anger. This is not to say that they do not feel emotions, it is that people with Asperger's feel extra emotions than any other "group" in the world. Identifying and expressing them in socially acceptable ways is what causes concern. To express your anger in an appropriate manner, you first need to be able to identify what underlying emotion you are experiencing. You need to find the root of the problem.

Anger can occur when a need is not being met or when others do not live up to our expectations. If people do not behave sensitively or considerately towards us when we expect them to, we can get angry. One of life's common upsets occurs when we allow the experience of external situations or the actions of another person to hurt us. If we do not allow ourselves to feel the pain and resolve the situation by discussing it, the pain can often lead to anger. If we repress the anger and the pain, we end up accumulating repressed feelings, which leads us to become angry more easily and often. This is not a healthy situation as it can cause damage to our health, as well as, personal relationships.

The medical profession has proved that when we live our lives under a high amount of stress, combined with a chronic build-up of anger, it can make us more susceptible to ailments such as diabetes, heart disease, insomnia and a weakened immune system. Often those close to us, also feel the impact of irrational and unrestrained anger. For the health and wellbeing of ourselves, and the people around us, it is important that we address the issue of anger management.

Anger management is not about preventing the emotion occurring, this is also not a healthy position because, it leads to repression and more extreme unforeseen emotional outbursts later. Instead it is about learning techniques that can enable you to work with anger in a more healthy way.

Recognizing the anger

The first step towards anger management is recognizing when we are angry. As well as our own unique signs of anger, there are common traits that occur when we experience anger. These include things like a tightened jaw, eyes wide open or constantly blinking, a sudden surge of energy in the body combined with an increased body temperature, or very cold in the case of cold rage.

As well as the common signs, become aware of your own body signals when you start to feel angry. When you begin to become aggravated, your body will relay signals and warning signs. Some people will bounce their knee, while others bounce their foot or bite their nails, etc. If you do not notice your body's signs of anger, then ask a friend or family member if they have noticed a body movement that you do when you get angry. If they have not noticed, ask them to pay attention to you the next time you get aggravated.

Many poker movies show body language subtleties. In the movie Maverick, Mel Gibson's character is a fantastic player because he learns everyone's signal, or "tell", when they are stressed, bluffing or excited because they have a winning hand. In the movie, "Rounder's", Matt Damon's character beats his opponent at the end of the movie by learning that his opponent's "tell" was how he played with his cookies. Another great TV show that teaches people about different micro-expressions is the show, "Lie to Me."

Common Signals:

1. Tensed Fist
2. Biting or picking at nails
3. Twirling or pulling at hair
4. Muscle Twitching
5. Playing or twirling a certain object
6. Bouncing knee or leg
7. Bouncing a foot

How to control your anger

The good news is- **you have control**! You can learn how to better navigate those feelings of anger. A common trait in people with Asperger's is the ability to switch from calm, to being infuriated very quickly. Considering how fast the Aspie brain works, it makes logical sense that when something happens, their thoughts would cycle around the occurrence raising the level of irritability to anger very quickly.

Anger that is out-of-control will hurt your relationships with loved ones, friends and colleagues. In the same respect, withholding your anger is not the answer either. Ignoring or denying your feelings of anger will build tension, which could cause your anger to elevate to rage later. Anger will eventually emerge, one way or another, so let us find some ways to manage anger in a healthy, constructive way without hurting or offending others.

Think First – SPEAK LATER

If you become involved in a heated discussion, refrain from saying the first thing that comes into your mind. These thoughts arise as a defensive reaction and do not resemble your true feelings. This saves you from feeling regretful later, which creates further stress. The best course of action is to allow time for everyone to calm down first. If possible, go for a walk, breathe deeply and allow the cortisol and adrenaline pumping through your veins to disperse. Punch a pillow. Scream into a pillow. Hug a pillow. Throw yourself on your bed. Massage your temples. Meditate.

When you and the other person have had time to calm down and have time to think about the situation without the veil of anger, then you are ready to sit down to talk. Both people should have a turn to speak and to listen to the other person. It is extremely important to not only listen, but to *hear* what is being said. Often disagreements arise from a misunderstanding or incorrect perception of what actually occurred. Do not spend the time when you are listening to prepare your next debate, invest in listening and the situation can be resolved, dissolving stress and negativity.

You can use specific phrases when you find yourself involved in conflict, which allows space for calm to develop. The parents in the TV series "Parenthood" state, "I hear you and I see you", and walk away from the other until they are calm. Once this has been achieved, they can discuss the situation from a better perspective resulting in a positive resolution for both sides.

If you feel anger arise when you are reminded to do certain tasks, such as taking out the garbage, you can choose to think differently about the situation. Being aware that you always have a choice is very helpful. You can say to yourself, or aloud if better, 'yes, this is my choice', or, 'I choose to take out the garbage now.' When people feel in control of their choices, when deciding to do what is expected of them, it leads to calmer feelings.

You can choose to create a positive outcome or choose not to do what is expected of you, potentially causing upset. "I choose to take out the trash and be in harmony with my spouse/parent" or "I do not enjoy taking out the trash, but I do not enjoy my spouse being unhappy, either." Remember, in all situations, you have a choice. The outcome always lies in how you react to a situation. That is empowering and important to remember.

A very wise crane operator that I know often uses the phrase, "Happy wife, Happy Life." Unlike, most of his construction coworkers, he is still married to the same wonderful wife 30 years later. He is often asked how he has remained happily married for so long and he smiles and just says, "Happy wife, Happy Life." You have the choice. Most of the time, your partner or parent will tell you what is expected. You have the choice to stand by your agreements or to let your partner or parent down. People count on one another and disappointment can quickly lead to anger. If you have trouble doing what is expected of you, consider making a chart to avoid confusion. Some people find it juvenile, but charts can be useful for everyone. When my children were old enough to do chores, I made a chart and added my husband's chores and mine. For the first time since we got married, he remembered to do his agreed chores. I no longer found myself struggling to take out the trash while pushing a baby in a stroller because he now had a visual reminder to do it. The bonus is he has a much happier wife. The result is a less stressed and much happier relationship. A happy partner likes to show their appreciation which adds to the overall harmony of the relationship.

Practicing forgiveness

We can often end up in a cycle of resentment when someone has done or said something to us that we did not like and we cannot let it go. Resentment develops when we continue to hold onto negative feelings about another or a situation and refuse to forgive. This then leads to more anger and more resentment; a vicious circle that also leads to ill health.

Forgiveness is not about accepting what the other person has done, or condoning their behavior; it is about choosing to stop holding onto something in the past and the negative emotion of resentment it brings. Your emotions are created, not by the other person involved, but from the thoughts and subsequent feelings that you have created from the situation. The power is always in your hand; choose to forgive so that you can feel better now and in the future. We all make mistakes, forgive and move forward.

If you are unsure of the process of forgiveness, many meditation mp3's can be downloaded from Amazon.com or iTunes. There are also excellent books devoted to the whole area of forgiveness, as it is a common block to happiness in so many people's lives.

Changing your mindset

Another suggestion is to practice changing the way that you think. By eliminating words from your daily vocabulary, such as 'never' and 'always' for example, you are training your mindset to become more optimistic. Using statements such as "I never have a good day" or "I am always late" are ways to justify anger but leave you with no option of improving the situation. Listen to your negative self-talk, identify what words and phrases you use daily which keep you stuck in a negative mindset. Choose to work on one at a time to eliminate these blocks to happiness.

Using relaxation techniques such as diaphragmatic breathing, meditation and physical relaxation techniques, like Tai-chi, Qigong, and Yoga, that we will discuss in chapter 7, will gradually lead to an overall decrease in anger levels.

When to Seek Professional Help

Anger is a natural emotion, but when it starts to spoil your work or personal relationships, then it is advisable to seek help. There is nothing wrong with seeking advice on how to manage your stress and anger. It makes sense for diabetics to see a nutritionist to learn healthier cooking and eating habits to regulate blood sugar levels; in the same way people struggling with anger issues seek help from a psychologist that specializes in Cognitive Behavioral Therapy to regulate anger levels.

According to the American Psychological Association (APA), individual and group cognitive behavioral therapy is scientifically proven to help control anger. The University of Chicago studies have shown that people's aggression, anger, hostile thinking and depressive symptoms had all decreased during therapy and in a three-month follow-up. Learning CBT techniques to control your impulsive anger issues can be enormously helpful; due to CBT's method of repeating positive behavior, the new pattern of thinking becomes ingrained in your mind resulting in changes in behavior. I have personally seen the benefits of CBT.

It is advisable that you see professional help if you display some of the following signs:

- Screaming (especially closely to someone's face)
- Hitting (hitting a pillow or other soft object is ok to constructively release built up tension)
- Throwing Things
- Coworkers/boss/H.R. meets with you about your demeanor at work
- Relationship problems (friends or a loved one feel like they're walking on eggshells)
- Frequent Arguments with people
- Harming yourself
- Engaging or threatening violence
- Driving Recklessly while angry

- Get annoyed with people easily
- Have trouble forgiving
- Seek revenge of people
- Say things that you regret
- Get into trouble with the law

Chapter 5 - Depression

It is important to note that the medical field is still unsure if depression automatically comes with Asperger's Syndrome or if the experiences and life struggles of having Asperger's lead to depression. Ultimately, the issue exists and needs to be addressed.

The DSM (Diagnostics Statistical Manual) defines depression as:

Five or more of the following criteria have been present during the same 2-week period and represent a change from previous functioning; at least one of the symptoms is either 1. depressed mood or 2. loss of interest or pleasure. **Note:** Do not include symptoms that are clearly due to another medical condition.

1. Depressed mood most of the day, nearly every day, as indicated by either subjective report e.g., feels sad, empty or hopeless or observation made by others e.g., appears tearful. **Note:** In children and adolescents, it can be an irritable mood.
2. Markedly diminished interest or pleasure in all, or almost all, activities most of the day, nearly every day, as indicated by either subjective account or observation from another.
3. Significant weight loss when not dieting or weight gain e.g., a change of more than 5% of body weight in a month, or decrease or increase in appetite nearly every day. **Note:** In children, consider failure to make expected weight gain
4. Insomnia or hypersomnia nearly every day.
5. Psychomotor agitation or retardation nearly every day, observable by others, not merely subjective feelings of restlessness or being slowed down.
6. Fatigue or loss of energy nearly every day.

7. Feelings of worthlessness or excessive or inappropriate guilt, which may be delusional, nearly every day, not merely self-reproach or guilt about being sick.

8. Diminished ability to think or concentrate or indecisiveness, nearly every day, either by subjective account or as observed by others.

9. Recurrent thoughts of death, not just fear of dying, recurrent suicidal ideation without a specific plan, or a suicide attempt or a specific plan for committing suicide

There are many reasons for depression but we will discuss the biological and environmental causes of depression.

Depression caused by a chemical imbalance

Sometimes the biological make up of a person is the cause of their depression. This is related to a chemical imbalance causing a lack of serotonin being produced.

Doctors have found that people suffering with depression have a smaller hippocampus. A smaller hippocampus means less serotonin receptors. Serotonin receptors are the calming chemical in the brain known as the neurotransmitter. The neurotransmitter is responsible for involuntary sensory perceptions, sleep and emotions including depression.

Serotonin allows communication between the brain and body. Another neurotransmitter, which is suspected to affect depression, is the neurotransmitter norepinephrine. People suffering with depression can have insufficient serotonin and norepinephrine levels. Dopamine is another neurotransmitter that involves movement, attention, learning and pleasurable sensations.

Many drugs increase dopamine levels in the brain. Drugs interfere with the function of neurotransmitters in the synapse.

Unfortunately, after prolonged drug abuse, the body slows down the production of dopamine because it becomes dependent on the person providing it through drugs, such as cocaine.

The antidepressant medications work in conjunction with the brains' biology, regulating these brain chemicals known as neurotransmitters, allowing for mood elevation.

Depression caused by past traumas

It is very important to recognize and deal with past emotional issues such as bullying or abuse, which is extremely common among the Asperger's population. Depression, in some ways, can be viewed as the lack of emotional expression. When we repress and hold onto repetitive negative thoughts and feelings, we become depressed.

One solution for this form of depression is to allow ourselves to feel those repressed emotions from the past in a conscious way. This can help us accept and then release them. It can be helpful to attend a counseling session or talk about what has happened with a trusted friend. Sometimes, allowing the feelings to emerge while doing physical exercise (such as jogging) can be a way to deal with uncomfortable feelings.

Cognitive and Dialectic Behavioral Therapy

One of the methods of treatment we have mentioned previously is Cognitive Behavioral Therapy (CBT). It is important to note that CBT is about finding solutions, unlike psychoanalysis that can take years of therapy sessions to see positive change; most patients see improvements within an average 16 sessions of CBT. The method is based on the fact that people form depressive, self-deprecating beliefs based on negative past experiences or detrimental statements deep in their unconscious. So people unconsciously form beliefs such as, "I can't do anything right" or "I'm worthless." Cognitive Behavioral Therapists work on eliminating these self-deprecating beliefs, showing them to be untrue.

Another form of CBT that is effective in helping Asperger's patients with depression is Dialectic Behavioral Therapy (DBT). Marsha Linehan created Dialectic Behavioral Therapy to treat both herself and her patients suffering with depression and suicidal thoughts. DBT teaches users how to handle life experiences more successfully by practicing four modules. The four modules are:

1. Distress Tolerance
2. Interpersonal Effectiveness
3. Emotional Regulation
4. Mindfulness

Distress Tolerance

Marsha Linehan states that DBT emphasizes the need to develop strategies on how to tolerate emotional pain skillfully. The ability to tolerate and accept distress is an essential mental health goal for at least two reasons. First, pain and distress are a part of life; they cannot be avoided or removed entirely from your experiences. The inability to accept this immutable fact itself leads to increased pain and suffering. Second, distress tolerance at least over the short term, is part and parcel of any attempt to change oneself; otherwise, impulsive actions will interfere with efforts to establish desired changes."

Linehan stresses the importance of the saying, "Acceptance of reality is not equivalent to approval of reality."

"The distress tolerance behaviors targeted are concerned with tolerating and surviving crises and accepting life as it is in the moment. Four sets of crisis survival strategies are taught: Distracting, self-soothing, improving the present moment and thinking of the pros and cons."

Interpersonal Effectiveness

This deals with learning how to communicate effectively with people while keeping your self-respect.

Check out this website for a more detailed view on the specific steps of handling Interpersonal Effectiveness -

It is common for CBT patients to complete assignments to try to prove or disprove personal belief statement and habits. Just like medication, the first one you try may not be a right fit for you; do not give up. Keep searching and trying until you find a therapist that works well for you, but keep in mind that CBT is built on the idea that a "sound therapeutic relationship is necessary for effective therapy, but not the focus." Therapists are more like a teacher or a guide helping you to help yourself. A good place to start is to ask your PCP doctor or review the list of doctors available through your insurance provider. There are some great websites providing reviews and directories of therapists such as the one listed on Psychology today and Psych Central.

Take the time to do your "homework", research the therapist before your first appointment. Ensure the person is a certified therapist and is knowledgeable about Asperger's Syndrome. If you do not feel comfortable with them, then move on to the next therapist on your list. You are in charge. You can quit therapy at any time and move on to the next therapist if necessary. Do not give up at the first hurdle; there is help available that will suit your needs. Find what works best for you. You deserve to be functioning at your emotional best. It may involve a journey of twists and turns, but you will feel like you have conquered a mountain when you begin master your emotions. The benefits of this liberating achievement will be worth the journey; you will reap wonderful rewards immediately and throughout your life.

Mindfulness

There has been a lot of research released recently into the positive effects of practicing Mindfulness in dealing with depression. It allows people to accept and tolerate the powerful emotions that they experience as part of depression.

The practice of Mindfulness is derived from the traditional Buddhist practice of being mindful of everything they do in each moment. In the context of DBT however, there are no religious or metaphysical concepts applied to the practice of mindfulness. Mindfulness within the context of DBT, teaches clients to pay attention to their present thoughts and feelings throughout the day, in a non-judgmental capacity. They are advised to watch the thoughts arise and fall away without attaching any significance to them. This allows one to live in the present moment, not attaching to past or future events, reducing the overpowering feeling of depression.

Medications

Many people do not want to begin taking medication for symptoms of depression. It is important to note that everyone has depressive times in his or her lives. However, when you are suffering with major depression it will affect not only your emotional and physical wellbeing but also those close to you. There is no reason to be embarrassed about taking medication for depression. This may be the best possible treatment route for you at this current time. It is simply helping to regulate a chemical imbalance in your body. Medication for depression combined with Cognitive Behavioral Therapy has been the best combination of therapy for people with Asperger's and depression. However, finding the right medication is not always an easy task. Everyone has different body chemistry, which is why many of these medications need to be tried and tested, until one that truly works well for you, is found.

If you need an increase in serotonin then a SSRI might help, but it can take up to six or eight weeks to determine if the effects of the medication are helpful for you. Sometimes a change in medication or an increase in the dosing is necessary. For some people they need an increase in serotonin and norepinephrine, in which case the SNRI or TCA medications will work better. For others, the best medication may be the use of Bupropion. Sometimes doctors will prescribe two medications from two different antidepressant classes. Consult a doctor to discover the best approach to relieving your depression. Most doctors will ask questions to determine if lifestyle changes can help alleviate some of your depression.

Chapter 6 - The Art of Empathy

Empathy is defined by the Merriam-Webster Dictionary as, *"the action of understanding, being aware of, being sensitive to and vicariously experiencing the feelings, thoughts, and experience of another of either the past or present; without having the feelings, thoughts, and experience fully communicated in an objectively explicit manner."* Neuro-typical adults often refer to empathy by using metaphors such as, *"put yourself in my shoes"* or *"try to see the situation through my eyes."*

Empathy can be difficult for a Neuro-typical person to express, but for those with Asperger's, it is a genuine struggle. This is in part because empathy requires the empathizer to decipher the body language of the person in addition to listening to what they are saying.

However, not everyone with Asperger's has difficulty with empathy, a certain percentage suffer from hypersensitivity. This is when people become super sensitive to the emotions of others. We will cover hypersensitivity later in the chapter.

The art of empathizing

Many people find it hard to empathize because they are not experiencing the issue themselves. However, the first step in empathizing with someone is to think of a personal past experience that has caused you stress or sadness. You do not have to have experienced the same circumstances as theirs; try to remember a time when you were struggling with something similar. Try to recall your thoughts and emotions at that time. Then listen attentively to the person.

Often the person seeking empathy just needs to be listened to, to feel understood and possibly just to vent about the situation at hand. If the person is aware that you have Asperger's, then they should not expect you to make eye contact. Keep in mind though, that you should stop what you are doing and listen intently; they need to feel validated. Validating someone's feelings is the act of making a person feel understood and respecting their feelings by allowing them to feel that way. Part of this is to make them feel like they have your undivided attention so they get a sense that you care about what they are going through.

As you listen to what they are saying, you need to try to be aware of their nonverbal expressions. If they are crying, then obviously they are sad. If they are crying and laughing then they are overtly happy. If they are clenching their fists, then they are angry, and so on.

Next, when they stop talking for a minute, you might want to say, "I am trying to empathize with you." Then ask, "Do you just need to vent? Do you want advice from me or some input into the situation?" Sometimes someone will just want you to listen and at other times, that person will want you to offer advice about the situation by trying to think of possible solutions.

The last step is often the most difficult; try to compare your past issue/experience with what the person is currently experiencing. At the same time, remember to keep them, not you, at the center of the conversation. Briefly mention your experience, but do not elaborate or remain stuck in your experience unless they ask you for specifics.

Lastly, never walk away; ask them if they feel better about the issue or mention that you hope this conversation eases some of their stress and anxiety.

Comments to avoid saying:

- I hope this never happens to me.
- I do not understand why you are feeling this way.
- Stop crying.
- Crying will not help.
- Are you finished yet?

The Steps for empathizing:

1. Think of a personal experience that made you feel frustrated or sad like the person that requires empathy.
2. STOP whatever you are doing and give them your full attention.
3. Look at the person's body language or nonverbal expressions.
4. State, "I am trying to empathize with you."
5. Ask, "Are you just venting or do you want me to help find a solution?"
6. Compare your experience to help you relate to how the person feels right now.
7. Do not get up or walk away until you have asked the person one of the following questions:
   "Do you feel better?"
   "Has this conversation helped?"

Hypersensitivity

We mentioned earlier in the chapter that some people with Asperger's become super-sensitive to the feelings of others.

Since the existence of hypersensitivity is a rather new "discovery," not much information is published on how to handle this overwhelming feeling. Currently, there are no medications available to calm the neurons that are being inundated with messages of empathy. This is why it is common for empaths to withdraw from society. Dr. Judith Orloff suggests that empaths need time alone to "decompress" from all that they "intuit and absorb." Orloff recommends setting "boundaries" as to how long and with whom you spend your time. She recommends having your own separate space and even suggests sleeping alone because empaths are known to have "energy fields blend with others during sleep, which can overstimulate empaths."

Another "empathy expert," Dr. Michael R. Smith, founder of Empath Connection, reassures highly sensitive people that negative energy can be avoided if you "learn how to quiet the mind so you have an awareness of when people infringe on your energy." Dr. Smith recommends meditations such as yoga and martial arts to connect the mind and body.

Phylameana Lila Desy writes in her article about "Hypersensitivity: What does it mean to be hypersensitive" that the highly sensitive person (HSP) will "learn which foods, scents and people cause symptoms of unease." She recommends diet modifications and avoiding perfumes and cleansers that are heavily scented.

Be aware which scents can be very calming or overwhelming for you. It is very important to pay attention to and keep a written record of what caused a negative reaction so you can avoid it in the future.

Chapter 7 – Emotional Mastery and the healthy lifestyle

We have covered many aspects of the emotional system so far with tips and suggestions for varying issues. However, an aspect that is often overlooked is the fact that though there are different methods to help you reduce the levels of anxiety and emotional distress in your life, there are other actions to undertake to help you feel more alive and happy.

In this chapter, we will discuss practical things that you can do to enhance your quality of living. These techniques really work, but they take some effort on your part to apply them in your daily life. You have already taken the first step towards positive change in your life by reading this book.

The key to emotional mastery really comes down to one major part of your being: your body. The wisdom of our body is often overlooked; for people with Asperger's there is often a commonality where we listen to our minds more than our bodies. Whether this is due to the condition or the fact that it is sometimes painful to be present in our bodies is not clear.

This chapter provides techniques that will help nourish your body and relaxation techniques suitable for providing some respite from your mind, allowing you to be present in your body.

Nutrition and Diet

There is a direct correlation to what you eat and how you feel and act. As an adult, you have the power to choose what to put in your body. If you are not getting enough vegetables in your diet because you prefer smooth foods due to an oral sensitivity, then consider puréeing vegetables or buying baby food containing these. If you enjoy cooking, perhaps try "The Sneaky Chef Cookbook" by Missy Chase Lavine, to incorporate a wider range of nutritious foods into everyday dishes. In "Deceptively Delicious: Simple Secrets to Get Your Kids Eating Good Food", by Jessica Seinfeld, she 'sneaks' pureed cauliflower into mashed potatoes and pureed carrots into popsicles.

Nowadays everyone has an awareness of the crucial importance of maintaining a healthy lifestyle, but for adults with Asperger's obstacles can get in the way. If you have depression, it does not help that the body increases its production of the stress hormone cortisol, which causes cravings and in turn usually leads to increasing weight. Eating a well-balanced diet can prove challenging for Aspies with sensory issues that have a limited diet; the use of herbs and organic vitamins can replace missing nutrients that you may not be receiving from your limited diet.

It is important to be aware of the choices you make in regards to your food consumption; the amount of artificial coloring, flavoring, genetically modified organism (GMO), hormones, high fructose corn syrup and preservatives can be high in certain foods. The human body can absorb these additives in moderation; however, the problem is that they are in such a vast amount of foods and condiments that people are absorbing these artificial substances into a body that is not equipped to properly dispose of them on a daily basis. DAN Doctors, Defeat Autism Now! from the Autism Research Institute, believe that autism is a biomedical problem that is, "*caused by a combination of lowered immune response, external toxins from vaccines and other sources and problems caused by certain foods.*"

Some of the major interventions suggested by DAN practitioners include:

- Nutritional supplements, including certain vitamins, minerals, amino acids and essential fatty acids
- Special diets, totally free of gluten (from wheat, barley, rye, and possibly oats) and free of dairy (milk, ice cream, yogurt, etc.)
- Testing for hidden food allergies, and avoidance of allergenic foods
- Treatment of intestinal bacterial/yeast overgrowth (with probiotics, supplements and other non-pharmaceutical medications)
- Detoxification of heavy metals through chelation (a potentially hazardous medical procedure)

Many people have praised the DAN doctors and have witnessed significant changes in the children that are under their care. Those who have tried the DAN interventions report increases in attention, focus, ability to complete tasks and overall calm behavior. Although there is still further research required, one thing is clear - the diets work when carried out correctly. In the book, 'Living Gluten-Free for Dummies', Danna Korn explains how gluten sensitivity and celiac disease can lead to, "behavioral manifestations" such as:

- Inability to focus or concentrate
- Attention deficit disorder (ADD) and attention deficit hyperactive disorder (ADHD) type behavior,
- Autistic and related behaviors

- Depression, bipolar disorder, schizophrenia and mood disorders
- Irritability, anxiety and lack of motivation

People with celiac disease or gluten sensitivity have trouble absorbing nutrients and produce an increase in stress hormones such as ACH and ACTH.

Filling our bodies with unnatural ingredients is unhealthy, yet the effectiveness of DAN interventions is still being debated due to a lack of medical studies. I, personally, have seen a marked improvement in a teen with Asperger's who changed her diet by eliminating dairy, chocolate, red 40 and yellow 6 (preservatives found in many processed foods in the US, they may be called something else in other countries).

Most people recommend that you eliminate one item at a time for two weeks to see if there are any improvements and then remove another item until you have your desired outcome. It is recommended that you test for allergies and sensitivities to know which foods and additives to eliminate based on what your body processes least effectively; certain foods and additives are triggers for people. It can take up to 72 hours to develop a reaction to something consumed, visit a professional for medical advice and determine which intervention is best for you.

Becoming gluten-free can be intimidating and overwhelming but there is a great website entitled, "Talk About Curing Autism", TACA, which provides lists of food, including the specific brands that you can eat and recipes that can be very helpful during this transition. It is encouraging to see the amount of food that is available.

If you do not have a gluten or dairy sensitivity, you might still want to consider a healthier way of eating, if you currently do not consume many nutritious foods. Other than the GFCF, (gluten free casein free), there are many alternative "diets" or ways of eating and cooking that are a healthier for your body. One "diet" that has received great reviews that I have tried personally is by Tosca Reno. It is a method of eating more natural and less processed foods. Tosca Reno has many books full of recipes and ideas; you will find helpful hints about how to replace sugar and use natural sweeteners like agave nectar and honey, etc. In addition to her books, she has a great website, Eat Clean Diet and online community.

Being around Positive People

Making and keeping friends can be difficult for people with Asperger's. However, a support system is essential. Consider joining a group or an online club. It is important to surround yourself with positive people.

Just as it is important for an alcoholic to avoid bars and drinking, it is as important for people that are stressed to avoid people and places that are negative. If you cannot find a local group to join, then consider joining an online community.

If you cannot find an online group that you would like to join, then you can start a group. Check out www.groupbox.com , they are a free service that enables you to start an online group. I have also joined groups using www.meetup.com.

They have countless groups to choose from ranging from cooking groups, chess groups, hiking groups, sensory related groups, anxiety groups, adults with Asperger's group, etc. Whether you join a group for support, to make friends or to enjoy a common hobby, there are many available; it is helpful to find people that share a common life experience, hobby or talent.

Relaxation Techniques

It is extremely important to learn relaxation techniques to help reduce stress and anxiety. Increased stress and anxiety increases the "fight or flight response." This occurs when the body prepares to fight or run, due to a perceived fearful event. Panic attacks trigger the "fight or flight response", which in turn increases blood flow up to 400%, rapid heart rate, high blood pressure and quickened breathing. According to the University of Maryland Medical Center, these reactions over time, raise cholesterol levels, disturb intestinal activities and depress the immune system. Finding effective relaxation techniques is beneficial to everyone's emotional and physical health.

> "In the mid-1970s, a Harvard cardiologist named Herbert Benson refers to changes that occur in the body when it is in a deep state of relaxation. These changes include decreased blood pressure, heart rate, muscle tension and rate of breathing, as well as feelings of being calm and in control. Learning the relaxation response helps to counter ill effects of the fight or flight response and over time, allows the development of a greater state of alertness. The relaxation response can be developed through a number of techniques, including meditation and progressive muscle relaxation. It is now a recommended treatment for many stress related disorders."

Dr. Herbert Benson has proven with over 150 medical studies that relaxation or meditative techniques have healing power, as long as the technique consists of two steps. The relaxation technique must include both the following:

1. A repetition of a sound, word, phrase or movement

2. The person must be able to set aside intruding thoughts.

Types of Relaxation

Autogenics

Also known as autogenic relaxation, or autogenic training, this is a form of self-hypnosis where visual imagery and body awareness are used in combination to achieve a deep state of relaxation before using affirmations to create changes in the person's behavior. This type of self-regulation was first created by Dr. Johannes Schultz of Germany and was further introduced worldwide by his student Dr. Wolfgang Luthe.

Qigong or Chi-Gong

According to the Qigong Institute, the word Qigong, pronounced, "chee gong", is a combination of two ideas: "Qi" means air, breath of life or vital energy of the body, and "gong" means the self-discipline skill of working, cultivating and balancing Qi. The art of Qigong consists primarily of the use of intention, meditation, relaxation, physical movement or posture, mind-body integration and breathing exercises. Practitioners of Qigong develop an awareness of qi sensations (energy) in their body and use their mind to guide the Qi for improving their health. Medical Qigong has been extensively studied scientifically more than any other alternative therapy and it has been shown to be a cost-effective therapy. Ultimately, Qigong is not about pursuit of excellence in form; rather, it involves experience through practice.

Diaphragmatic Breathing

Diaphragmatic Breathing (or relaxation breathing) is breathing that involves using your diaphragm correctly to strengthen the diaphragm muscles, decrease your breathing rate and decrease oxygen demand. The diaphragmatic breathing technique involves putting one hand on your heart and the other on your belly just below your rib cage. You slowly and gently breathe in through your nose pushing out your belly and then slowly contract your stomach muscles bringing your belly back in while exhaling through pursed lips.

Jogging (or other cardiovascular exercise)

As discussed in the relaxation techniques section of this chapter, the "fight or flight response" increases blood flow in the body but it also increases adrenaline. Due to this physical reaction, many health professionals recommend exercise to alleviate the extra adrenaline that is produced from the body's reaction. Have you ever heard someone use the phrase, "run it off?" This phrase refers to running until all of the excess adrenaline in the body has decreased to a normal level.

Meditation

According to www.webmd.com meditation, *"consists of the silent repetition of a word, sound, or phrase, perhaps one that has special meaning to you, while sitting quietly with eyes closed for 10 to 20 minutes. This should be done in a quiet place, free of distractions. Sitting is preferred to lying down in order to avoid falling asleep. Relax your muscles starting with the feet and progressing up to your face. Breathe through your nose in a free and natural way. During a meditation session, intruding worries or thoughts should be ignored or dismissed to the best of your ability, by focusing on the sound, word or phrase. It is OK to open your eyes to look at a clock while you are practicing, but do not set an alarm. When you have finished, remain seated, first with your* eyes closed and then with your eyes open and gradually allow your thoughts to return to everyday reality."

Passive Muscle Relaxation

Passive Muscle Relaxation is a type of relaxation where you imagine your muscles are all fully relaxed. Because there is no muscle tension created in this type of muscle relaxation, it is safe for all people.

Progressive Muscle Relaxation

This is a type of relaxation that involves tensing your muscles for ten seconds and then relaxing them for 30 seconds. However, it can raise blood pressure so do not perform progressive muscle relaxation without consulting a doctor. According to the www.helpguide.org the steps to progressive muscle relaxation are:

- Loosen your clothing, take off your shoes and get comfortable.
- Take a few minutes to relax, breathing in and out in slow, deep breaths.
- When you feel relaxed and ready to start, shift your attention to your right foot. Take a moment to focus on the way it feels.
- Slowly tense the muscles in your right foot, squeezing as tightly as you can. Hold for a count of 10.
- Relax your right foot. Focus on the tension flowing away and the way your foot feels as it becomes limp and loose.
- Stay in this relaxed state for a moment, breathing deeply and slowly.
- When you are ready, shift your attention to your left foot. Follow the same sequence of muscle tension and release.
- Move slowly up through your body, contracting and relaxing the muscle groups as you go.
- It may take some practice at first, but try not to tense muscles other than those intended.

Progressive Muscle Relaxation Sequence:

The most popular sequence runs as follows:

1. Right foot*	6. Left thigh	11. Right arm and hand
2. Left foot	7. Hips and buttocks	12. Left arm and hand
3. Right calf	8. Stomach	13. Neck and shoulders
4. Left calf	9. Chest	14. Face
5. Right thigh	10. Back	

* If you are left-handed, you may want to begin with your left foot instead.

Tai Chi

A series of movements, performed either very slowly or quickly to help move the body's chi (energy). According to www.umm.edu:

> *"There are various perspectives on how tai chi works. Eastern philosophy holds that tai chi unblocks the flow of qi. When qi flows properly, the body, mind, and spirit are in balance and health is maintained. Others believe that tai chi works in the same way as other mind-body therapies and there is ample evidence that paying attention to the connection between the mind and the body can relieve stress, combat disease, and enhance physical wellbeing."*

Tai chi has three major components -- movement, meditation, and deep breathing.

- **Movement** -All of the major muscle groups and joints are needed for the slow, gentle movements in tai chi. Tai chi improves balance, agility, strength, flexibility, stamina, muscle tone and coordination. This low impact, weight-bearing exercise strengthens bones and can slow bone loss, thus preventing the development of osteoporosis.

- **Meditation** -Research shows that meditation soothes the mind, enhances concentration, reduces anxiety and lowers blood pressure and heart rate.
- **Deep breathing** -Exhaling stale air and toxins from the lungs while inhaling a plentitude of fresh air increases lung capacity, stretches the muscles involved in deep breathing and releases tension. It also enhances blood circulation to the brain, which boosts mental alertness. At the same time, the practice supplies the entire body with fresh oxygen and nutrients.

Yoga

Yoga is an ancient art of harmonizing the body, mind and spirit using eight "limbs", two of which include asana (postures) and pranayama (diaphragmatic breathing). According to the Harvard Health Publications April 2009 publication, studies prove that yoga is an effective form of treatment for stress and anxiety.

In addition, the regular practice of both asana and pranayama leads to greater internal sensitivity, which can allow students to detect the first glimmer of an anxiety or panic attack and respond with yogic tools that might head off the problem. The earlier you can intervene, the greater the likelihood of its effectiveness.

There are many types of yoga, but the most commonly practiced and researched is Hatha yoga. This originated in India in the 15th century, giving a slow-paced gentle workout. The focus is on breathing and meditation.

Knitting:

Knitting is a hobby that includes using knitting needles to weave together yarn to create items of clothing. In 2007, research done at Dr. Herbert Benson's "Harvard Medical School's Mind/Body Institute proved that knitting induces the relaxation response and lowers heart rate on average by 11 beats per minute" because of the rhythmic clicking sound of the knitting needles. Another positive body response found in this study was a decrease in blood pressure.

Conclusion

We hope that you benefitted from the topics discussed in "Emotional Mastery" and picked up some positive guidelines to help you understand your emotions and to implement to improve how you live your life.

The most important thing now is that you put some of these actions into practice. Remember, it all starts with recognizing the emotions you are feeling. Then by understanding the triggers that occur in your life, you will feel empowered, knowing that you have choices in how you respond to any situation.

Longer-term health and well-being will also depend on a change in diet and lifestyle. We have mentioned the dietary recommendations and relaxation techniques in this book because they are proven methods in producing positive change. If you commit to a change in the way you think, feel and live, you will experience big changes in your emotional well-being.

Find some relaxation techniques that you enjoy and develop a plan about how you will implement these into your life. Not everyone likes knitting for example but perhaps you feel more attracted to yoga or jogging. Choosing an alternative practice of behavior that you enjoy doing will help you adhere to your new plan, creating a greater chance of success at mastering your emotions.

We realize as we started writing this book together that there is actually so much we could have included in the subject of emotional mastery. There is a full range of emotions, social interactions and contexts we could have included but in the end, we wanted to focus on the chief concerns from readers. Based on feedback received from running The Asperger's Test Site, we have covered most of the major areas that adults with Asperger's struggle with on a daily basis.

We will hopefully be releasing further publications to address issues like relationships, confidence issues, making friends and succeeding in the workplace. If there are other topics you feel you would like to hear about or if you have specific feedback about this book, please contact us on the Asperger's Website or send us an email us at info@AspergersTestSite.com.

We would be really grateful if you could review the book on Amazon.com. We do appreciate your feedback.

For more helpful information on Asperger's Syndrome you can subscribe to our newsletter at:
http://www.aspergerstestsite.com/aspergers-newsletter

Please feel free to check our website for a range of free articles that you may find interesting and helpful.

Works Cited

American Psychiatric Association. 30 Apr 2012. Major Depressive Episode. 15 Aug 2012.
<http://www.dsm5.org/ProposedRevisions/Pages/proposedrevision.aspx?rid=427>

Anestis, Michael D. "Dialectical Behavior Therapy Skills Part 3: Emotion Regulation." 07 April 2009. Florida State University. 18 Sept 2012.
<http://www.psychotherapybrownbag.com/psychotherapy_brown_bag_a/2009/04/dialectical-behavior-therapy-skills-part-3-emotion-regulation.html >

Anxiety and Panic Disorders Health Center: Post Traumatic Stress Disorder. 2005-2012. Webmd. Sept 2012.
<http://www.webmd.com/anxiety-panic/guide/post-traumatic-stress-disorder?page=2 >

Anxiety Disorders. 2 Nov 2010. National Institute of Mental Health. 12 Aug 2012.
<http://www.nimh.nih.gov/health/publications/anxiety-disorders/complete-index.shtml>

"Anxiety in Adults with an Autism Spectrum Disorder." 9 July 2012. The National Autistic Society. Sept 2012. <http://www.autism.org.uk/living-with-autism/understanding-behaviour/anxiety-in-adults-with-an-autism-spectrum-disorder.aspx>

"Asperger Syndrome Fact Sheet." National Institute of Neurological Disorders and Stroke. May 2007/22 Aug 2012. National Institutes of Health. Sept 2012. <http://www.ninds.nih.gov/disorders/asperger/detail_asperger.htm >

Autistic Spectrum Disorders: Fact Sheet. Sept 2012 <http://www.autism-help.org/family-suicide-depression-autism.htm>

Burby Jr., James. Personal Interview about Dan! Doctors. 20 Aug 2012.

Burgin, Timothy. "Anxiety." Yoga Basics. 2001-2012. Sept 2012. <http://www.yogabasics.com/learn/anxiety.html.>

Chakraburtty, Amal. WebMD Health News. 03 Feb 2006. The Cochrane Review. Aug 2012. <http://www.webmd.com/anxiety-panic/guide/20061101/best-ways-to-ease-anxiety-disorders >

Depression Health Center: Causes of Depression. 2005-2012. WebMD, LLC. Sept 2012. <http://www.webmd.com/depression/guide/causes-depression>

"Depression (Major Depression)." 10 Aug 2012. Mayo Foundation for Medical Education and Research. 15 Sept 2012. <http://www.mayoclinic.com/health/antidepressants/MH00071>

Desy, Phylameana lila. "Hypersensitivity: What does it mean to be hypersensitive?" 2012. About.com. 22 Sept 2012. <http://healing.about.com/od/empathic/a/hsp.htm>

Dickens, SD. "How Knitting Can Relieve Stress and Lower Blood Pressure." 12 Aug 2012. HubPages. Sept 2012. <http://sd-dickens.hubpages.com/hub/How-Knitting-Can-Relieve-Stress>

Dietz, Lisa. "DBT Lessons: Emotion Regulation Overview." 2003-2012. DBT Self-Help. 20 Sept 2012. <http://www.dbtselfhelp.com/html/overview2.html>

Dietz, Lisa. "DBT Skills List." 2003-2012. DBT Self-Help. 21 Sept 2012. <http://www.dbtselfhelp.com/html/connecting_skills.html>

Diseases & Conditions: Positions to Reduce Shortness of Breath. 15 Aug 2008. Cleveland Clinic. Aug 2012. <http://my.clevelandclinic.org/disorders/chronic_obstructive_pulmonary_disease_copd/hic_positions_to_reduce_shortness_of_breath.aspx>

"Frequently Asked Questions: What is Qigong?" 2004-2012. Qigong Institute. Aug 2012.
<http://www.qigonginstitute.org/html/FAQ.php >

Gaus, Valerie. "Cognitive-Behavioral Therapy for Adult Asperger Syndrome." 6 Jul 2012. Psychcentral. 17 Sept 2012.
<http://psychcentral.com/lib/2009/book-review-cognitive-behavioral-therapy-for-adult-asperger-syndrome>

Goldberg, Joseph. Anxiety & Panic Disorders Health Center: Mental Health and Hypnosis. WebMD. 05 June 2012.
<http://www.webmd.com/anxiety-panic/guide/mental-health-hypnotherapy >

Hockenbury, Don H., and Sandra E. Hockenbury. *Discovering Pyschology Fifth Edition*. New York, NY: Worth Publishers, 2011. Print.

Hooper, James F. and John M. Grohol. Pysch Central. 01 June 2010. Pysch Central. Sept 2012.
<http://psychcentral.com/disorders/sx25t.htm>

"Inerpersonal Effectiveness." CBT Recovery. 19 Sept 2012.
<http://www.cbtrecovery.org/interpersonaleffectiveness.htm>

Kaim, Nomi. Asperger's Association of New England. 2011. AANE. <http://www.aane.org/asperger_resources/articles/miscellaneous/aspergers_depression.html >

Kay, Heidi. Personal Interview about DBT solutions. 23 Sept 2012.

Korn, Danna. *Living Gluten-Free For Dummies*. Hoboken: John Wiley and Sons, 2010. Print.

Lawson, Jake. "Self-Affirmations." 28 Nov 2011. Demand Media Inc. Sept 2012. <http://www.livestrong.com/article/15086-self-affirmations/>

Lodge, Meredith. Personal Interview about DAN! Doctors. 21 August 2012.

"Making Sense of Dialectical Behaviour Therapy." 2012. MIND. 18 Sept 2012. <http://www.mind.org.uk/help/medical_and_alternative_care/dialectical_behaviour_therapy#DBT >

Markram, Henry and Tania Rinaldi and Kamila Markram. "The Intense World Syndrome-An Alternative Hypothesis for Autism." 2007. US National Library of Medicine, National Institutes of Help. 19 Sept 2012. <http://www.ncbi.nlm.nih.gov/pmc/articles/PMC2518049>

Massachusetts General Hospital. 2012. The Benson-Henry Institute for Mind Body Medicine. Sept 2011. <http://www.massgeneral.org/bhi/about>

McCall, Timothy. Yoga Journal. 2012. Cruz Bay Publishing. Aug 2012. <http://www.yogajournal.com/for_teachers/2390 >

Miller, Tara. "100 Natural Ways to Overcome Anxiety." USPharmD. 09 Dec 2008/updated 2012. USPharmD. Sept 2012. <http://www.uspharmd.com/blog/2008/100-natural-ways-to-overcome-anxiety/>

Morin, Amy. Livestrong. 8 Aug 2011. Livestrong. Sept 2012. <http://www.livestrong.com/article/511084-types-of-therapy-for-aspergers/#ixzz24s4shGIA>

NACBT Online Headquarters. 05 April 2007. National Association of Cognitive-Behavioral Therapists. 20 Sept 2012. <http://nacbt.org/whatiscbt.htm>

Nauert, Rick. "SSRIs Effective for Depression." 26 Aug 2009. Pysch Central. 15 Sept 2012. <http://psychcentral.com/news/2009/08/26/snris-effective-for-depression/7987.html>

Ogbru, Omudhome. "Bupropion, Wellbutrin, Wellbutrin SR, Wellburin XL, Zyban" 1996-2012. Medicine Net, Inc. 28 Sept, 2012. <http://www.medicinenet.com/bupropion/article.htm>

Orloff, Judith. "Relationship Secrets for Highly Empathic People. 30 June 2010. Huffington Post.com, Inc. 15 Sept 2012. <http://www.huffingtonpost.com/judith-orloff-md/relationship-advice-relat_b_628549.html>

Psychology Today. 2002-2012. Sussex Directories, Inc. 23 Sept 2012. <http://www.psychologytoday.com/basics/cognitive-behavioral-therapy>

"Relaxation Techniques." 1997-2012. University of Maryland. A.D.A.M., Inc. Sept 2012. <http://www.umm.edu/altmed/articles/relaxation-techniques-000359.htm>

Robinson, Lawrence and Melinda Smith and Jeanne Segal. "Obsessive-Compulsive Disorder (OCD): Symptoms and Treatment of Compulsive Behavior and Obsessive Thoughts. June 2012. Helpguide. Sept 2012. <http://www.helpguide.org/mental/obsessive_compulsive_disorder_ocd.htm#signs >

Rudy, Lisa Jo. About.com: Autism Spectrum Disorders. 22 July 2009. Medical Review Board. Aug 2012.

<http://autism.about.com/od/alternativetreatmens/f/dandoc.htm
>

Sammy. "Feb 5th & 7th Classes." Dialectical Behavior Therapy-
University. 09 Feb 2007. DBT-U. 22 Sept 2012. <http://www.dbt-
u.com/category/emotion-regulation>

Santa Maria, Cara. "Anxiety vs. Stress: What's the Difference?" 15
Dec 2011/20 Sept 2012. Huffington Post. 25 Sept 2012.
<http://www.huffingtonpost.com/2011/12/15/anxiety-stress-
difference_n_1152590.html >

"Selecive Serotonin Reuptake Inhibitor." 23 Sept 2012. Wikimedia
Foundation, Inc. 28 Sept 2012.
<http://en.wikipedia.org/wiki/Selective_serotonin_reuptake_inhi
bitor >

Smith, Melinda and Ellen Jaffe-Gill. Social Anxiety Disorder and
Social Phobia: Symptoms, Self-help, and Treatment. June 2012.
Helpguide. Sept 2012.
<http://www.helpguide.org/mental/social_anxiety_support_symp
tom_causes_treatment.htm#common>

Smith, Michael R. "Are You an Empath? What is an Empath?" 30
Sept 2012. <http://empathconnection.com>

Soraya, Lynne. "Asperger's Diary: Life Through the Lens of
Asperger's Syndrome." 12 Sept 2010. Sussex Directories, Inc. 26

Sept 2012. <http://www.psychologytoday.com/blog/aspergers-diary/201009/aspergers-pain-perception-and-body-awareness>

Stress Management. "Types of Relaxation Techniques." 2008 Stress Management Health Course. <*http://stresscourse.tripod.com/id38.html.*> Sept 2012.

Sunnen, Gerard V. Ozonics International. 2006. Ozonics International LLC. Sept 2011. <http://www.triroc.com/sunnen/topics/hypn&anxiety.htm>

Svahn, Krister. Sahlgrenska Academy. 06 Feb 2012. University of Gothenburg. Sept 2012. <http://www.sahlgrenska.gu.se/english/news_and_events/news/News_Detail/depression-common-among-young-adults-with-asperger-syndrome.cid1062430>

Szalavitz, Maia. "Asperger's Theory Does About-Face." 14 May 2009. Toronto Star. 17 Sept 2012. <http://www.thestar.com/article/633688>

Tillman, Jane. "Distress Tolerance Handout I: Crisis Survival Strategies." 1993. Guilford Press. 27 Sept 2012. <http://www.janetillman.com/Distress_Tolerance.pdf>

Tull, Matthew. "Ways of Coping with Anxiety." 14 May 2009. Medical Review Board. Sept 2012. <http://ptsd.about.com/od/selfhelp/tp/anxietycoping.htm>

WebMD. "Antidepressants: Myths and Facts About SSRIs. 2005-2012. WebMD, LLC. 20 Sept 2012. <http://www.webmd.com/depression/ssris-myths-and-facts-about-antidepressants>

"Yoga For Anxiety and Depression." Harvard Health Publications. April 2009. Harvard Medical School. Sept 2012. <http://www.health.harvard.edu/newsletters/Harvard_Mental_Health_Letter/2009/April/Yoga-for-anxiety-and-depression>

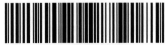

24564385R00051

Made in the USA
San Bernardino, CA
02 October 2015